Everyday dentistry for the cat and dog

John G A Robinson
BDS

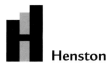

Henston

Henston

Henston
A Division of Veterinary Business Development
Olympus House
Werrington Centre
Peterborough
PE4 6NA

Telephone: +44 (0) 1733 325522
Facsimile: +44 (0) 1733 325512

Designed and produced by Veterinary Business Development Ltd

ISBN 1 85054 187 6

© 2002 Henston Ltd

Reprinted 2006

Price £7.50

Acknowledgements

All photographs are the property of and are reproduced with permission from John G A Robinson

® Veterinary Business Development Ltd

About the author

John G A Robinson BDS

John qualified as a dentist from Kings College Dental School, London in 1984 and then worked in general dental practice for six years.

His interest in veterinary dentistry began in 1988 but it was not until 1992 that it became his full-time occupation. Having taken a year out to travel, serendipity took John to San Francisco where he met Dr Michael Floyd. The following three months spent with Michael Floyd were the steepest part of the learning curve in the transition to animal dentistry. The last ten years have been spent in pursuing any and all openings and requirements connected to companion animal dentistry.

John has been the Course Organiser of the British Veterinary Dental Association since 1995, which mainly involves running postgraduate courses and developing undergraduate teaching at the English Veterinary Schools. He lectures and teaches veterinary dentistry internationally.

John also treats clinical cases, both referral and first opinion, at The Village Animal Hospital in Caterham, Surrey and at The Bishops Veterinary Surgery in Hatfield, Hertfordshire. He works with veterinary organisations and companies to promote and develop animal dentistry.

Contents

Foreword

We humans take teeth for granted and notice them only when they cause us pain. Yet for the veterinary practitioner, dentistry can be a very interesting and rewarding area.

In human dentistry nowadays, all efforts are concentrated on restoration and preservation. Those times when the brutal removal of a stubborn wisdom tooth was the stuff of slapstick comedy – but certainly no laughing matter in real life – are, thankfully, over. Advanced materials, new instruments and improved techniques have helped to make this transition; and the majority of these instruments and techniques are also available to the veterinary dental surgeon.

I am delighted that John G A Robinson, an accomplished expert in human dentistry as well as animal dentistry, has been willing to share his wealth of knowledge and expertise with us. Although dentistry is still not fully developed in all veterinary practices, I feel that this handbook should help to take the subject an important step away from the mere pulling of teeth, towards a more sophisticated service.

As a publication for general practice, the Henston Veterinary Guide *Everyday dentistry for the cat and dog* is not intended to be a fully comprehensive textbook. It is more a useful training and reference tool for the practitioner and provides a solid foundation for the provision of dental care for small animals. It ranges from anatomical features to a description of instruments, and covers all the important aspects for the practice dental team.

I would like to thank Penelope Lyons, David Weaver and Mike Fleming for their invaluable contributions to the successful production of this publication.

Peter Mueller

Introduction

Ten years ago, I made the transition to dentistry for companion animals instead of for people. Then, animal dentistry was a neglected area with no formal teaching available and a 'learn in the saddle' attitude. Animal dentistry has since improved greatly, but there is still a considerable gap between the current, accepted knowledge and the dental care provision for our pets.

My dream is a time when all pets can receive good basic dental care and so have pain-and-infection-free mouths. Recognising when there is a dental problem and dealing with it in a simple and predictable way, often by tooth extraction, is the foundation to attaining a healthy mouth. At present, this goal has to take priority over more advanced dentistry geared towards keeping teeth.

The road ahead may be daunting but progress is made by each step and, when we look back, we can take comfort in the distance already travelled. I hope this book will enable me to escort those in the front line of animal care, a good few steps along the journey of veterinary dentistry.

1 Anatomy and physiology

Head anatomy in the dog and cat

A working knowledge of the anatomical features in proximity to teeth is important in understanding their inter-relationship in disease and treatment. Avoiding iatrogenic damage requires awareness of neighbouring structures.

The inferior alveolar canal

This canal runs through the body of the mandible in close proximity to the apices of all the mandibular teeth. It contains the neurovascular bundle, which includes the sensory trigeminal nerve, supplying the teeth and distal areas. When extracting mandibular teeth, care must be taken not to instrument beyond the root end. In the cat, a root can easily be pushed into the canal.

Branches exit via the mental foramina. The main mental foramen is close to the apex of the lower canine tooth – remember this when performing a surgical extraction or interpreting radiographs of this tooth.

The nasal cavity

The maxillary teeth (except the molars) are in close proximity to the nasal cavity. The bone between the medial side of the upper canine tooth and the nasal cavity is egg-shell thin and can easily be disrupted during tooth extraction or lost if there is chronic pathology at the site (e.g. periodontal disease). The palatal root of the upper carnassial tooth also has an especially close relation to the nasal cavity and infection at this root can track into the nose. Care should be taken when extracting this root not to displace it, by inward pressure, into the nose.

The infra-orbital neurovascular bundle

This bundle runs through the maxilla in close proximity to the root apices of the upper carnassial tooth and emerges through the foramen, level with the caudal root of the third premolar tooth, and then runs superficially across the maxilla. It is important to remember this structure when raising buccal gingival flaps, as when performing a surgical extraction of the carnassial tooth.

The orbit

The upper second molar is in close proximity to the base of the orbit. This association is relevant with infection. When extracting this tooth, care must be taken not to slip off the caudal aspect and allow the elevator to penetrate caudal to the maxilla.

The tooth

A tooth may be considered as a calcified peg but general orthopaedic principles are inapplicable. When considering or handling a tooth, a different approach is required from bone. Teeth have negligible capability for repair.

Components of the tooth and gingiva (Figure 1) are discussed below.

Enamel

The enamel thickness in cats and dogs is a fraction of that in human teeth. It is completely formed before tooth eruption. The enamel forms the tough outer shell of the crown but if lost or defective it is not a major concern. Exposed dentine is sensitive to temperature changes (only when drinking cold water or panting in dogs). After about a month, the dentine becomes sclerotic and the sensitivity ceases. Enamel provides a smooth surface but when damaged or defective becomes more plaque-retentive.

Pulp–dentine organ

The bulk of a tooth is made of dentine. When a tooth erupts the root is incompletely formed and more dentine is laid down to complete the length and then close the apex. The pulp canal is a chamber (or canal) in the tooth. There is a layer of cells, the odontoblasts, at the interface of the

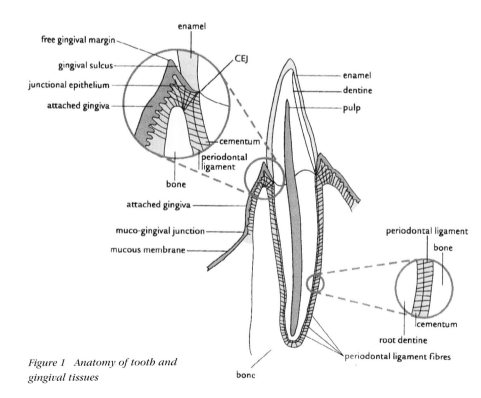

Figure 1   Anatomy of tooth and gingival tissues

pulp and the inner surface of the dentine. Each cell has a long tapering process that extends through the dentine, normally almost to the outer surface. Thus, the dentine is not solid but is rather like a mesh, due to the thousands of tubules per square millimetre. The odontoblasts produce more dentine, which thickens the dentine of the crown and root, with a corresponding reduction in the size of the pulp canal. This occurs rapidly in the first year after eruption and then more slowly. If there is external stimulation, after exposure of the dentine surface, the odontoblast processes retreat and fill the tubule with dentine – the dentine is now said to be sclerotic.

Pulp

The pulp is not merely 'the nerve'. It is a complete connective tissue including all usual components such as the lymphatics. The innervation of the pulp gives sensitivity to heat and cold. The stimulus is passed through the odontoblast processes.

The other sensation from the pulp is pain. The pulp is a delicate tissue that becomes inflamed in response to insults such as thermal trauma and bacterial ingress. The pulp is contained in a finite space and so can not expand when inflamed, resulting in severe pain.

Cementum

The root dentine is covered by a thin layer of bone-like substance called cementum. The Sharpey fibres of the periodontal ligament insert into the cementum to make a strong attachment.

Periodontal ligament

The periodontal ligament is the soft tissue sandwich between the bony socket and the tooth root. It is a matrix of fibres supported by a connective tissue. The innervation of the periodontal ligament gives the sensation of pressure or load on the tooth and also pain from damage or infection of these tissues.

The gingiva

Gingiva (or gum) refers to the specialised epithelial tissues, along with their connective tissue base, that are around the teeth. Sub-groups include the junctional epithelium, the free gingiva (marginal gingiva), and the attached gingiva.

Junctional epithelium

The body's epithelium is a continuous barrier to the external environment except where the teeth protrude through. The junctional epithelium forms the internal surface of the gingiva and interfaces with the tooth surface to maintain a seal against the tooth. Normally, the junctional epithelium attaches to the enamel at the base of the tooth crown. The junctional epithelium is thin and the surface cells have hemidesmosomes, akin to mini suckers, on their surface which make a relatively weak attachment to the tooth. There is no mechanical interlock but merely an abutment.

Free gingiva

Even in clinically healthy gingiva, the cells of the junctional epithelium do not maintain an attachment right up to the reflection at the gingival margin. This means that the tip of the gingiva is not attached and is referred to as the 'free gingival margin'. A groove (gingival sulcus) is formed between the free gingival margin and the tooth. This can be as deep as 3 mm at some teeth in larger dogs. It is considered normal, but only when there is a healthy band of junctional epithelium attached to the crown.

Attached gingiva

Externally there is a band of thick, heavily keratinised epithelium. On the buccal aspect of the teeth, the attached gingiva extends from the gingival margin to the freely mobile mucous membrane. The two tissues are demarcated by the line called the mucogingival junction. The attached gingiva is firmly bound down to the bone and teeth by fibres running through the connective tissue. The attached gingiva forms a zone of tough tissue that is not dislodged by the large forces exerted on it in function. The width of the attached epithelium should be at least 3 mm.

Dental formulae and tooth eruption times

Figures 2 and 3 represent the deciduous and permanent dental formulae in the dog and cat

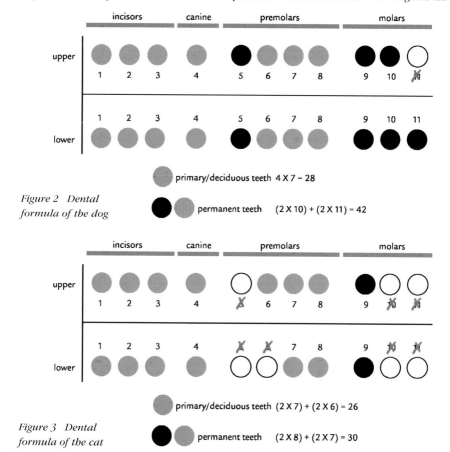

Figure 2 Dental formula of the dog

Figure 3 Dental formula of the cat

respectively. The uncoloured circles represent teeth that are absent compared with the full mammalian formula. All deciduous teeth are replaced by a permanent successor.

Eruption times are quite variable; Figures 4 and 5 show common time ranges in the dog and cat respectively.

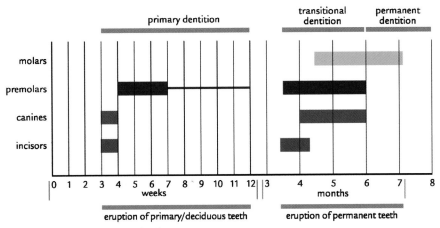

Figure 4   Eruption times in the dog

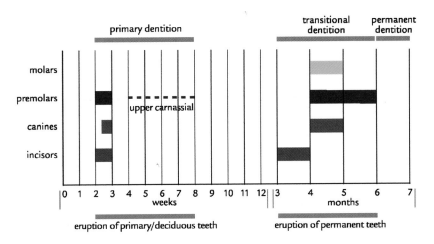

Figure 5   Eruption times in the cat

2 Oral examination

Initial visual examination

An oral examination is part of every physical examination. The initial oral examination is performed on the conscious animal and is limited to visual inspection, although possibly with some digital palpation. Having looked at the entire face, the mouth is first examined by gently holding it closed and just retracting the lips to look at the soft tissues and buccal aspects of the teeth. This is also the optimum time to examine 'the bite' (occlusion), checking whether or not the mouth can close completely and that no trauma is being caused by any tooth impinging on soft tissue. Finally, the mouth is gently opened by:

- placing a thumb and finger on the alveolar crest caudal to the canine teeth of each jaw and encouraging the mouth open

- for the mandible in cats, placing a finger on the lower incisors.

In large dogs, the pits and fissures in the molar teeth should be checked for tooth decay (caries).

When fractured teeth are discovered at the initial oral examination, the options of extraction or root canal therapy can be offered.

Definitive oral examination

The definitive oral examination can only be carried out under general anaesthesia. Then the teeth can be cleaned and dried (using compressed air) for good visibility and also probed. The entire soft tissues of the mouth are screened. The teeth are examined in detail in a systematic manner and abnormalities are recorded on a dental chart (see page 8). As each tooth is examined, so is its associated gingiva, periodontal attachment and bony support.

Any missing tooth is noted on the chart, usually by drawing a circle over its picture. The tooth crowns are checked for abnormalities; the common ones being fractures, wear (attrition), discoloration, resorptive lesions (especially in cats) and tooth decay (in dogs).

Where a tooth is fractured, it should be determined whether or not the pulp canal has been exposed. The site can be probed forcefully to look for an opening. A fine seeker probe (see page 48) is useful to find small openings. Where there is a communication between the pulp canal and the oral environment, bacterial ingress will cause a pulpitis and subsequent necrosis so necessitating treatment.

Gingivitis

The amount of bleeding resulting from running a blunt-ended periodontal probe gently around the gingival sulcus is assessed at each tooth. The gum margin is assessed for visual signs of inflammation. The highest score of these two indices is allocated as the gingivitis score (Table 1).

Table 1 Assessing gingivitis

Gingivitis score	Gingivitis index (modified from Loe & Silness indices)
0	normal or healthy gingiva
I	slight inflammation: slight redness and/or oedema delayed, slight bleeding on probing
II	moderate inflammation: redness, oedema and glazing bleeding on probing
III	severe inflammation: marked redness and oedema profuse bleeding on probing

Periodontal pocket depth

To assess and monitor periodontal disease, the pocket depths are measured, using a periodontal probe (see page 48). The degree of periodontal involvement and loss of attachment varies from tooth to tooth and also at different sites around each tooth. The pocket depth is the most important parameter in determining the prognosis and the treatment required in periodontal disease.

The greatest pocket depth is measured on both the buccal and the lingual aspect of every tooth. The periodontal probe is inserted behind the gingival margin and slid down the tooth root until, with only a few grams of pressure, the gingival attachment is felt. The probe is then moved around the tooth with the tip running along the bottom of the pocket. Abnormal pocket depths are recorded against their related position on the dental chart.

The clinical pocket depth is the measurement from the gum margin to the attachment. When there is gingival hyperplasia, an element of false pocket is created. The true amount of attachment lost is the distance from the edge of enamel or cemento–enamel junction (CEJ) to the tissue attachment on the tooth root.

The dental chart

A large amount of information results from the dental examination and is recorded on the chart in pictorial or notation form. At its most basic, it should record teeth that are already missing and teeth that need to be extracted along with the reason why. Ideally, all abnormalities should be recorded.

A completed chart is a legal record that can be referred to:

- during treatment – to ensure that all the extractions are performed, periodontal pockets can be relocated and treated
- at post-treatment discharge – to inform the owner what was done and the condition of the teeth
- at any time and by any person in the practice – for information relating to the mouth at a specific date.

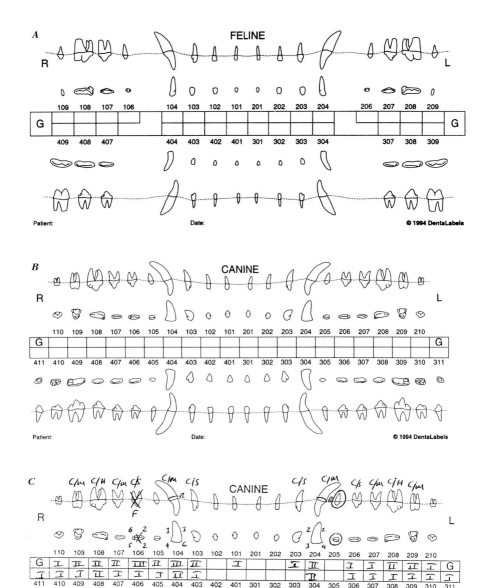

Dentalabels: A feline dental chart; B canine dental chart; C completed dental chart

8

Intra-oral radiography

Small dental films can be used inside the mouth to give high-definition images without the superimposition of structure on the contra-lateral side of the head.

Equipment

The equipment needed for intra-oral radiography is listed in Chapter 9 (page 48).

When do you need a dental radiograph?

Intra-oral radiography is indicated when additional diagnostic information is required for the structures below gum level (i.e. the roots and their bony support).

Common clinical situations that require a radiograph include the following.

1 Confirming whether or not a tooth pulp is non-vital by examining the periapical region of a tooth (the periodontal ligament space and the bone at the end of the root) for rarefaction. This is indicated in a tooth that is fractured, discoloured or has sustained trauma.

2 Identifying the problem when a tooth extraction is not progressing as expected – abnormal root curvature, ankylosis.

3 Assessing root remnants (including fractures during extraction) for size, shape, number, integrity and position. Also as a check that removal was complete.

4 Detection and evaluation of tooth root and bony fractures.

5 Confirmation that a tooth is missing rather than un-erupted (ectopic) or partly remaining. Buried teeth may have associated infection or give rise to cysts.

6 Assessing the extent of root resorption when extracting teeth with feline odontoclastic resorptive lesions. Also detecting root lesions.

7 Assessing the amount and pattern of bone of bone loss and remaining support of teeth in periodontal disease.

Techniques for intra-oral radiography

The normal principles of radiography all apply, but there are some practical differences compared to usual veterinary radiography:

- the non-screened film requires comparatively high exposure settings (using a veterinary machine and a normal film focal distance (FFD), an average setting would be 70 kV and 50 mA)

- the film packet contains a lead foil backing and thus has a specific side to face the beam (the packet is marked)

- placing a L or R marker would cover much valuable film area so there is an orientation dot in one corner.

The smallest size of film that will include the entire area to be examined is used; this allows the best possible positioning. The film is placed inside the mouth in such a way as to be as close to and as nearly parallel to the structures to be examined as possible. The film is held in position by placing some packing to hold the film the against the tooth but without bending the film. Screwed-up paper towel makes ideal packing.

Parallel technique

Parallel placement is only possible for mandibular teeth that are caudal to the symphysis (Figure 6).

The animal is placed in lateral recumbence with the side to be radiographed uppermost. The film is placed lingual to the premolar or molar to be radiographed and is then gently pushed ventrally to get the lower edge of the film level with the inferior border of the mandible. With the film held parallel to the subject, the X-ray beam is positioned perpendicular to both.

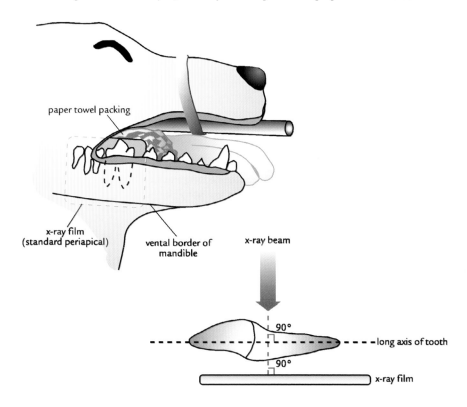

Figure 6   Intra-oral radiography: parallel technique on lower carnassial tooth

The bisecting angle technique

When radiographing teeth, other than the posterior mandibular teeth, it is not possible to place the film parallel to the subject. The film is still placed inside the mouth behind the subject tooth, at the smallest possible angle to the long axis of the subject (Figure 7).

If the X-ray beam were to be directed at 90° to the film, the image would be shortened. If the beam were to be directed at 90° to the long axis of the tooth, the image would be elongated. To achieve an image that is the same proportions as the subject, the bisecting angle technique

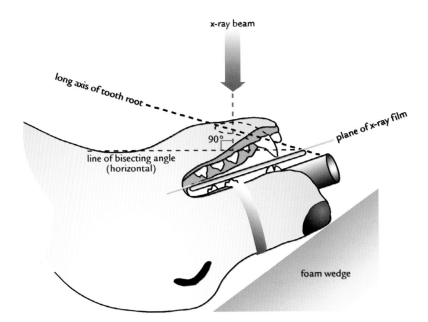

x-ray beam

long axis of tooth root

plane of x-ray film

90°

line of bisecting angle
(horizontal)

foam wedge

Figure 7   Intra-oral radiography: bisecting angle technique on lower canine tooth

is employed. An imaginary plane is visualised half-way between the plane of the film and a plane through the long axis of the tooth (i.e. at the bisecting angle) and the X-ray beam is directed at 90° to this plane.

Two tongue spatulas can be used to visualise the planes outside the mouth and so aid the positioning of the beam. It is very useful to have a mental image of the normal orientation, length and morphology of the tooth roots. A common problem is to miss the apex of a tooth, especially the canines, by poor estimation of length or position.

The advantage of a dental X-ray machine is that the machine head is very manoeuvrable and can be positioned around the animal's head. However, when using a veterinary machine with a beam that is limited to a vertical direction, the animal is placed in one of the following suitable positions:

- sternal recumbence for maxillary incisors
- lateral or sternal recumbence for maxillary canines, premolars and molars
- dorsal recumbence for the mandibular incisors and canines.

The head position is then adjusted to make the bisecting angle plane absolutely horizontal. The head is held in place by packing.

The canine teeth can be viewed latero-medially or rostro-caudally, depending on the reason for examination. Sometimes (e.g. when checking for root fractures), it is best to use both.

The bisecting angle technique can be used when an occlusal film (or small cassette) is placed across the tops of the teeth (on the occlusal plane). The film is easy to hold in place by closing the mouth, and its angulation is easy to see.

3 Periodontal disease: cause and effect

Periodontal disease (gum disease) is not a single disease but rather a spectrum of plaque-associated diseases with common factors. Adult-onset periodontal disease is the most common category and the general term 'periodontal disease' is assumed to refer to this form unless stated otherwise. Periodontal disease is the most common disease in cats and dogs. Indeed, it is so common in cats and dogs that all individuals should be considered at risk until proven otherwise.

Periodontal disease is an inflammatory and destructive condition affecting the support tissues of the teeth (the periodontium). It is not like other diseases in so much as there is not a cure but only a moderation of cause and effect. Controlling periodontal disease requires an individually tailored and lifelong management programme.

Dealing with periodontal disease is frustrating because it is a never-ending battle between plaque and the host. The management of the disease (plaque control by home care and treatment) aims to reduce the insult from plaque and aid the host response. Preventing plaque from gaining the upper hand is very difficult in the more prone individuals.

The progression of periodontal disease is a complex process in which many factors interplay. A huge amount is known about the process of adult-onset periodontal disease but many key factors are still unknown. Research to advance our understanding of this disease in humans, cats and dogs is ongoing. A working knowledge of the aetiology and pathogenesis of periodontal disease is required in order to understand how to make prevention and treatment of the condition effective and so achieve real and lasting benefits.

Normal gingiva

The clinically healthy gingiva appears as uniform pink in colour, except when there is black pigmentation, and is without any area of increased redness. It forms a firm knife edge against the teeth with no sign of oedema. There is no bleeding if the gums are probed or brushed.

Plaque

Plaque is the fundamental cause of periodontal disease and other oral disease. It is a soft, sticky, whitish accumulation on the surfaces in the mouth and especially the teeth. It has the consistency of a paste. Plaque is not easily rinsed from the tooth but can be dislodged by light mechanical scraping such as in tooth brushing. It is a similar colour to teeth, so is not easily visible. Plaque can be made clearly visible by applying a disclosing solution to stain it and then rinsing the excess solution from the teeth to leave the highlighted plaque. The disclosing solution can be any food dye; erythrosine is the one commonly used. In animals, disclosing is best done by swabbing the dye on with a cotton bud or similar applicator.

Plaque development

Immediately after a tooth crown is cleaned to bare enamel it becomes coated with saliva and normal commensal bacteria. Some of the bacteria produce long-chain polysaccharides that form a matrix to bind plaque. More bacteria accumulate on the surface to increase the thickness of plaque; this is possible as teeth provide a static, non-shedding surface. Plaque has other components such as dead cells and food substrates.

As plaque becomes mature, the micro-environment in the deeper parts favour a shift from a majority of gram-positive aerobes to gram-negative anaerobes, which are thought to be more harmful. The metabolic products and toxins produced by the bacterial plaque cause an inflammatory response in any soft tissue that is in close contact, initially the gingival margin.

Plaque will form without any food passing through the mouth as all the necessary components are already present. However, plaque accumulates more rapidly when sticky, high-carbohydrate foods are eaten.

Plaque is not a haphazard accumulation but a structured 'biofilm'. The structure protects the bacteria within from antibacterial agents: 50 to 100 times the normal application concentration of antibiotic would be necessary to be effective.

Calculus

Calculus is also known as tartar and scale. The terms are interchangeable; the one that is understood by the pet's owner should be used. Calculus itself may not be harmful but its surface is very rough and porous so plaque is always harboured both on the surface and within. With a base of calculus, plaque can not be completely removed even by tooth brushing. Calculus strongly adheres to the tooth and can only be removed by scaling techniques.

Calculus development

Saliva and gingival crevicular fluid have high levels of minerals, which calcify plaque. Calculus can form very quickly – less than 48 hours after the start of plaque accumulation.

Gingivitis

Gingivitis is the initial response to the plaque on a nearby tooth surface (Figure 8, overleaf). Gingivitis is inflammation of the gingiva which, by definition, is totally reversible once the cause is removed. When the gum margin is inflamed, the gingival sulcus becomes deeper; the base of the sulcus is then more hospitable to anaerobic bacteria. The flow rate of crevicular fluid, a gingival transudate, is increased.

Typical gingivitis is not at all painful. There are specific conditions that have an associated gingivitis that is painful but periodontal disease is not one of them. The degree of gingivitis can be graded using the modified Loe & Silness indices (page 7).

When there is a constant presence of plaque on the teeth, the gingivitis can not resolve and becomes established or chronic, and may remain in this state for several years. Then, at a certain point, the condition can change into periodontal disease. Typically, in cats and dogs,

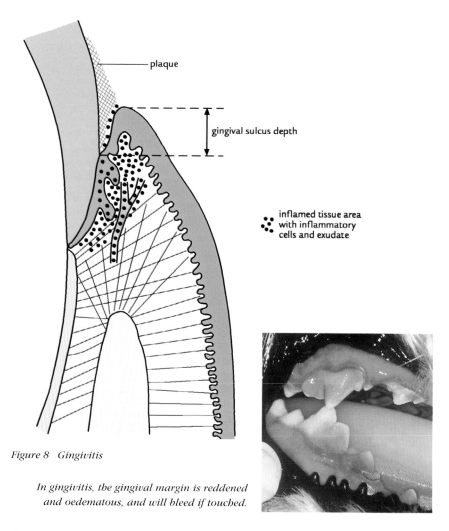

plaque

gingival sulcus depth

inflamed tissue area
with inflammatory
cells and exudate

Figure 8   Gingivitis

*In gingivitis, the gingival margin is reddened
and oedematous, and will bleed if touched.*

this occurs at about three or four years of age. It is not understood what factors cause the
transition. Gingivitis is a necessary precursor to periodontal disease but gingivitis does not
always become periodontitis.

Smaller dogs and cats, especially pure-breds, develop a periodontitis that starts at a younger
age and tends to be more rapidly progressive.

Adult-onset periodontal disease

At a certain stage, for reasons that are not understood, the host response to irritation from
plaque changes. The response, which is mainly under genetic control, changes from simple
inflammation to one that involves breakdown of host tissues in the area of chronic

inflammation. In some ways, it can be likened to a frustrated healing or foreign-body response. There is breakdown of the fibres that attach the gingiva, and of the bone forming the tooth socket (Figure 9). The gingival attachment to the tooth (junctional epithelium) migrates from the crown onto the root (in an apical direction) in an attempt to remain attached to a 'healthy' surface. Migration of the junctional epithelium results in the formation of a periodontal pocket. The destruction of the attachment and support tissues of the tooth progresses in periods of activity interspersed with periods of dormancy. Over time, more and more support is lost until the tooth becomes loose and may eventually fall out. The body has thereby expelled the problem (plaque) by sacrificing the tooth.

Once the support tissues have been destroyed, the changes are irreversible. The aim of treatment is to prevent or slow further destruction. When periodontal disease becomes more advanced, the anatomical changes form a local environment that aids the harbouring of plaque and calculus formation. As a result, the rate of progression of periodontal disease gathers momentum and treatment becomes more difficult. Deeper periodontal pockets are more difficult to instrument and maintain in a plaque-free condition.

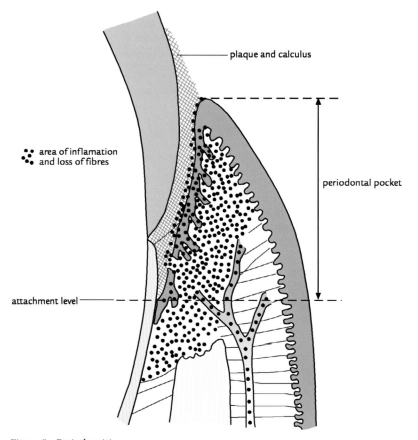

Figure 9   Periodontitis

The main objective in treatment is to enable optimal plaque control by altering the local environment. This is mainly by removal of the plaque-retentive calculus. When an area is made plaque free, the inflammation of the soft tissues resolves and there is some shrinkage of the gingiva in healing. This is seen as gingival recession. Both processes result in some reduction in pocket depth.

When there is deep pocketing and little residual bone support, disease progression can not be halted and the best option is tooth extraction.

Rate of progress of periodontal disease

The cause of the periodontal disease is plaque, but the pattern and rate of progress of the disease depends on the host response. The major factor determining host response is the animal's genetic programming. It is accepted that, in general, pure-bred cats and dogs are more prone to periodontal disease than cross-breeds. Certain breeds are more prone than others (e.g. Abyssinian cats are more prone than Siamese cats).

Other factors influencing the progress of periodontal disease are discussed below.

Immune status

Immune-compromised animals are likely to show a more rapidly progressive and severe periodontal disease. This is due to an impaired host response.

In cats with viral infections (e.g. FIV or FeLV), the difference may be so noticeable as to be an alerting sign of viral disease. Animals suffering from systemic diseases (such as diabetes or hypothyroidism), animals on long-term steroid therapy, and debilitated animals will be all be immune-compromised.

Severe malnutrition also causes more rapid periodontal disease but this is an extremely rare occurrence among pets.

Body mass

A rule of thumb is that the less the body mass, the greater the risk of periodontal disease. The risk for a cat is comparable to that for a dog of the same size. It is not certain why this is so, but the smaller dental anatomical entities mean that an equivalent amount of destruction in periodontal disease is more significant. There is also the 'critical bone mass' hypothesis, which is uncertain, but obviously smaller animals have less alveolar bone mass forming the tooth sockets.

Hormonal influence

In humans, female hormones have a huge influence in periodontal disease. This is why pregnant women and nursing mothers qualify for free dental treatment. The effect of hormones in cats and dogs has hardly been studied.

Diet

The diet is often thought to be the major factor in periodontal disease, whereas it actually plays only a minor role. Diet does influence the rate and type of plaque accumulation: sticky foods and those high in short-chain carbohydrates are likely to result in greater plaque accumulation. Without plaque, there is no gingivitis or periodontal disease. The amount of plaque needed to cause disease varies between individuals. In some cases, a small amount of plaque can result in a rapidly progressive and advanced periodontal disease; in others, heavy calculus and plaque accumulation may cause only a mild gingivitis.

Self-cleansing

Generally, too much importance is placed on the cleaning of the teeth from normal function (self-cleansing). There is an assumption that wild animals feeding on a natural diet have far fewer gum problems. In fact, wild animals commonly suffer from periodontal disease and, if it is to a lesser degree, many factors other than – or in addition to – the physical properties of the diet may be responsible.

Removal of some plaque occurs by the action of a chewed object (food or toy) sliding over the tooth surface. Tough objects can dislodge calculus. Less plaque, which also means less calculus formation, makes the mouth appear cleaner and smell less badly. However, the shape of teeth means that parts of the crown are not touched in the chewing action: the tooth surface close to the gum margin is not cleaned as the bulge of the crown deflects the chewed object. Build up of plaque at this site, close to the gingiva, is where it is most harmful.

There are foods, edible treats and other products available that have been designed with physical properties to maximise their tooth cleaning ability. Studies show these do reduce overall plaque and calculus levels. What is not proven, is how much clinical benefit this produces in terms of disease reduction. This is not to dismiss the benefits of these products, but the plaque control achieved is a fraction of that achieved by brushing the teeth. And even good tooth-brushing may not provide sufficient plaque control to prevent periodontal disease in the highest-risk individuals.

Stagnation areas and plaque-retentive factors

Tooth crowding, missing teeth, misaligned and rotated teeth, malocclusion, gingival recession or gingival hyperplasia all result in stagnation areas. The environment thus creates traps where plaque is protected from dislodgement by function or tooth cleaning. Plaque accumulation may accelerate periodontal disease.

Plaque-retentive factors are surfaces to which plaque can better adhere and become more difficult to remove by tooth cleaning or function. Examples are calculus, scratched teeth, fractured teeth, enamel defects and exposed root cementum.

Periodontal disease aggravating other diseases

It has been shown that scaling or extracting teeth with periodontal disease results in a bacteraemia. In deep and inflamed periodontal pockets the lining epithelium can be ulcerated and thus allow bacteria and bacterial toxins to enter the underlying inflamed and very vascular tissues and then the systemic circulation. In a site of advanced periodontal disease, the gingiva and tooth may become quite loose and the movement from chewing probably facilitates bacterial ingress.

There is a strong index of suspicion that in advanced gum disease a bacteraemia may occur many times a day, and to a greater level as more teeth have more advanced periodontal disease. At present, it cannot be said that this is the primary cause of disease at other organ sites but it can be presumed to be an aggravating factor. Renal disease and diseases involving endothelial damage are those of most concern but any disease site or area of compromised tissue may be affected.

Severe periodontal disease

Periodontal disease is largely not at all painful. Pain may result from tooth mobility or a periodontal abscess at a site with very advanced periodontal disease. The movement of a markedly mobile tooth in function will tear at the remaining gingival attachment and cause pain. In cats especially, a tooth just hanging on by gum attachment can make the animal almost anorexic but once the tooth is lost, normal eating resumes.

The amount of infection present in advanced periodontal disease can become so severe as to result in pyorrhoea (pus running from the gums). This has to significantly compromise general health.

No tooth should be allowed to deteriorate to advanced stage periodontal disease but should be extracted at an earlier stage once it is realised disease control is not possible.

4 Periodontal disease: home care

Regular plaque control and clinical dental treatments have to go hand in hand, if periodontal disease is to be effectively managed. Without adequate home care to maintain oral hygiene, all the benefits of performing a 'scale and polish' will last merely a matter of weeks.

Tooth brushing

Tooth brushing is the single most effective method of plaque control. It is simply mechanical removal of plaque and soft calculus. Today, people do not question that they should brush their own teeth every day. It is accepted as the mainstay in dental care. Periodontal disease in dogs is known to be the same disease process as in humans, and it is likely to be the same or very similar in cats. The conclusion should surely be that the same methods of disease control apply. Brushing a pet's teeth should be the same established habit.

Daily brushing establishes a routine and plaque is removed before it begins to harden (calcify) into calculus. The most important place to clean is at the gum line and gingival sulcus: this is where plaque is protected from removal during chewing (due to the contour of the tooth crown) and where it is in close proximity to soft tissue.

Selecting a toothbrush

There is no industry standard for tooth-brush hardness. A soft brush is not as effective in dislodging the plaque and will soon deform from its proper shape. A hard brush does not conform to the tooth surface contours and so does not clean recessed areas well. Hard brushes may also be abrasive. A medium brush should be employed.

Common sense would suggest that the gums of a dog are not more sensitive than those of people. The same type of quality brush should be used for pets as for humans. Choose the size of toothbrush according to the size of the pet:

- cats and miniature/toy breeds of dog – use the small, short-bristled CET® puppy brush (this is the same as the small end of the double-ended pet toothbrush)
- small to medium dogs – use a child's toothbrush
- medium (over approx. 10 kg) to large dogs – use an adult's toothbrush.

Toothpaste

Using toothpaste on the toothbrush gives only a slight increase in efficacy of plaque removal.

The main function of a pet toothpaste is to encourage pet co-operation by having an enjoyable flavour. This is especially important in cats, but can be counter-productive in some dogs as they like the taste so much they try to eat the brush. Malt flavour is liked well. Strong mint-flavoured toothpaste should be avoided as it seems to be unpleasant for most animals, perhaps even giving a burning sensation.

There are toothpastes specifically formulated for animal use. One brand contains a natural enzyme system, which although it does not have proven clinical benefits does have theoretical benefits and is non-harmful.

It is not advisable to use a toothpaste designed for humans. These may contain ingredients that are harmful when swallowed by a pet. For example, fluoride has proven benefits in combating tooth decay, which is why it is present in most human toothpastes. There is no indication for animals to have fluoride, and ingestion of it (especially chronic ingestion in cats) may lead to significant side-effects.

Techniques for tooth brushing

The goal is to brush all the buccal (outer, cheek-side) surfaces of the teeth each day. Ideally, the lingual (inner, tongue-side) surfaces should also be brushed but this is impractical except with very co-operative animals and a competent owner. There may be some cleansing action of the lingual surfaces by the tongue.

A technique for dogs

Prepare the tooth brush by applying the toothpaste and pushing it down into the bristles. Hold the dog's muzzle with the left hand to keep the mouth almost closed. Raise the upper lip with a thumb or finger of the left hand and insert the brush, at the corner of the lips, inside the cheek. Begin at the back of the mouth with the upper teeth, and brush all the outer surfaces of the teeth inside the cheek. The gum margin of the lower teeth can be brushed by just allowing the mouth to open slightly but not enough to enable the dog to chew the brush. Continue by brushing the teeth toward the front of the mouth up to the canine teeth. Change the left hand position on the muzzle to be able to lift the lip on the other side. Brush in the same way on the opposite side. Finish by brushing the incisors. The direction of brushing is less important than thoroughly brushing teeth in the order described.

A technique for cats

Raise the head by placing the right hand under the chin. With the left hand, stroke over the top of the head and drag the thumb or index finger over the lips to pull the lip corner (commisure) backwards and slightly upwards. This will create a slot between the lips which exposes the buccal surface of all the teeth. The cat's head is kept still by holding with the palm

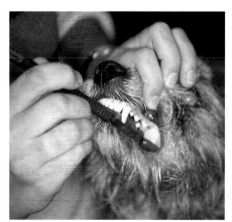

Dog having teeth brushed

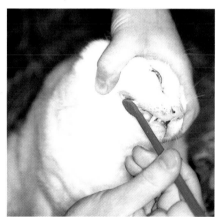

Cat having teeth brushed

on top of the head, the thumb and index finger tips on the lip commisures under the cheek bones and the other fingers on the back of the neck.

The bristles of the CET® puppy brush can be inserted through the slot between the lips while the head of the brush remains outside. The cheek teeth are cleaned with a horizontal motion and the canine teeth with a vertical motion.

Acceptance

Some animals (especially puppies) will not initially accept normal brushing or the owner may find the technique difficult. In either case, use the following gradual approach:

- use just a finger, perhaps with some pet toothpaste, to rub the outer (buccal) surfaces of the teeth
- next try a finger toothbrush (for dogs) or a cotton bud (for cats)
- finally, use a toothbrush to brush a few teeth behind the canines and increase the number of cheek teeth brushed as acceptance is gained (time tolerance will be increased)

Always give a treat or reward after home care for positive reinforcement.

In dogs that are trained sufficiently to accept control by the owner, over 90% should accept tooth brushing at any age. Starting to brush soon after the permanent teeth have erupted, around six months of age, will gain maximum prevention and also help with acceptance by the animal.

Cats are much more difficult animals in which to achieve acceptance of tooth brushing but greater success can be expected if the habit is established at a young age (beginning as a kitten). As cats are very prone to periodontal disease, the need for tooth brushing is great. Tooth brushing should be attempted for all cats but efforts stopped if the cat absolutely refuses.

Gingival bleeding

Tooth brushing results in bleeding when there is any area of gingivitis. This bleeding is not associated with pain but it is often misunderstood by pet owners who then cease brushing. The bleeding is an indicator of gingivitis and will reduce as plaque levels are reduced. After a week of daily brushing, the gingivitis should be markedly improved; absence of gingivitis shows that the plaque control is adequate. The standard of oral hygiene required to prevent gingivitis varies between individuals. Total resolution of gingivitis will not be achieved when there is calculus as some plaque will remain.

Chemical anti-plaque agents

The gold standard for chemical anti-plaque agents is chlorhexidine. Chlorhexidine has good broad spectrum antibacterial activity and is also effective against some viruses and fungi. Chlorhexidine is very safe with no significant side-effects. It has the property of substantivity, which means that it binds to the oral surfaces and is released in active concentrations for up to 12 hours.

Specific preparations of chlorhexidine are available for oral use in veterinary cases as solutions or gels. To achieve maximum benefit, the agent is applied liberally to cover the required area. Combining it with some mechanical cleaning to disrupt the plaque and debris will make chlorhexidine more effective.

If the standard of tooth brushing is insufficient to give adequate plaque control, using chlorhexidine gel instead of tooth paste is recommended. The chlorhexidine has only to work on the residue not removed by the mechanical cleaning.

Chlorhexidine applied topically, as a spray or simple coating with no mechanical cleaning, has about two-thirds the anti-plaque effect compared to thorough tooth brushing. Topical chlorhexidine can be used to promote healing of superficial oral lesions.

Other chemical anti-plaque agents are not as effective as chlorhexidine and have no additional advantages. Therefore, they are not considered here.

Putting brushing into action

Until recently, the idea of brushing a pet's teeth would have been regarded as strange. Now, the idea is generally accepted but only a minority of owners are actually brushing their pet's teeth. For tooth brushing to become a reality, owners need to be motivated and taught how to perform the task. They need to be educated in cause, effect and management of gum disease. Once owners realise the importance of plaque control, they are likely to feel that the effort is worthwhile.

Some motivational benefits are:

• no more bad breath (halitosis) or 'dog's breath'

• a healthier pet with possibly a greater life expectancy

• keeping the teeth for longer

• reducing the need for veterinary dental treatment and the associated expense.

In addition to motivation, owners have to be shown how to perform home plaque control for their pet. When demonstrating the technique, it is better not to do it perfectly on a trained animal but on the pet in question. Ask the owner to try out the technique so as to demonstrate what they can do. Some owners will find it easy. When an owner is not as willing, not so good at handling their pet or has a difficult pet, it will take longer to achieve the best possible results. In these cases, the owner's ability needs to be assessed with plenty of help and encouragement until the routine is successfully established. Reminders may be required to prevent a lapse in tooth brushing.

The benefits of chewing

Some people think that forceful chewing gives immense benefits in reducing periodontal disease and maintaining healthier teeth. Other people, including some experts, think that chewing has negligible benefits. The evidence is mainly anecdotal with insufficient scientific data available to support either view.

The cleansing action of chewing and its limitations in plaque reduction are discussed on page 17. There may be other ways in which chewing has beneficial effects. The physiological exercise of chewing may be beneficial to the periodontal ligament and the bone of the tooth socket.

It makes sense to promote whatever benefits can be obtained but at the same time to ensure safety. Whatever is chewed should not have the potential to harm in either its original form or once chewed. Many objects can be harmful to the mouth and teeth or when swallowed. Objects that are harder than teeth – bones, stones, hooves and artificial bones – should not be given. These can fracture teeth and are the main cause of slab fractures of the upper carnassial teeth in dogs. The greatest benefits are from tough objects that will yield and distort thus giving better tooth contact (compared to solid objects that only make contact with the most prominent aspect of the tooth).

Dogs derive much enjoyment from chew toys, the use of which should be encouraged as long as the toys are safe. Safe rubber toys and rawhide strips make good treats. Cats are not as interested in chew toys and have to be encouraged to chew with chewable foods and edible treats.

Summary

The goal in home care is to achieve sufficient plaque control for the individual. A high standard of tooth brushing is the ideal way of achieving this. Any level of brushing is for the good and short comings can be supplemented by other methods of plaque reduction (chlorhexidine and chewy treats). The owner should not be given the impression that their efforts are not worthwhile if they can not brush well. They should be encouraged to reach the best level of plaque control that is practical for them and their pet.

5 Periodontal disease: treatment

The treatment of periodontal disease is ongoing plaque control (home care) combined with clinical dental treatment at appropriate times. Prevention is better than clinical treatment. Prevention is achieved by establishing and continuing adequate plaque control. Early intervention requires simpler treatments and has a better long-term prognosis when followed up with appropriate home care. The rational of all treatment for periodontal disease is to make the oral environment optimal for plaque control.

'Doing a dental' is a rather general term for dental treatment. Professional periodontal therapy (PPT) is the treatment for periodontal conditions carried out under general anaesthetic. The main components of PPT are:

- scaling supragingivally and subgingivally (above and below the gum line)
- root planing
- polishing
- minor periodontal surgery
- tooth extraction.

The endeavour of the first three items has been nicknamed 'gum gardening' and is a thankless task if not maintained with home care.

Even when it is known that home care will not happen to any appreciable level, there are still reasons for performing clinical dental treatment. A proper assessment of the severity of the periodontal disease is gained by a complete oral examination under anaesthesia. Plaque retention is reduced by gross calculus removal and other plaque retention factors can be reduced (e.g. the removal of gingival hyperplasia). The ultimate treatment that safeguards the animal against the harmful effects of periodontal disease is tooth extraction. In established periodontal disease, aggressive selection of teeth for extraction will avoid the harmful effects of more advanced disease.

Health and safety

Certain precautions are necessary for any dental treatment under general anaesthesia.

Airway protection

It is necessary to protect the animal's airway from ingress of fluids and solid debris such as tartar or tooth fragments. Power scalers and dental drills spray large volumes of water into the mouth.

A throat pack protects against solid pieces, but cannot be relied on to stop all fluid. Fluids will run past a pack, along the outside of the endotracheal (ET) tube, and be directed into the trachea. In all dental treatments, a cuffed ET tube is necessary to seal the trachea. The throat pack must be frequently removed and wrung out. It should be attached to a highly visible object, which stays outside the mouth, to reduce the risk of forgetting to remove the pack before recovery.

When the animal is turned over while under anaesthetic, it must be done with the legs passing underneath the body. This way, the head will tip downwards and the mouth will drain out. If the animal were rolled over on its back, any fluids in the mouth would enter the throat.

Operator safety

Power scalers disturb the plaque in the mouth and create a bacterial aerosol. This will travel about two metres and hang in the air for several hours. All surfaces in that zone should be considered contaminated. The operator and anyone else within a two-metre radius should wear a good surgical face mask to prevent inhalation of large numbers of bacteria. Use of the drill and other instruments also disturb the oral bacteria but to a lesser degree.

It is recommended to clean the mouth with chlorhexidine solution and a tooth brush after the oral examination and before any treatment. This dramatically reduces the bacterial load in the mouth.

Wearing glasses is also recommended throughout dental treatment, especially when using any powered instruments, to protect the eyes from any flying calculus, tooth fragments, polishing paste or contaminated fluid spray.

Professional periodontal therapy

A suggested approach in PPT is:

- record calculus deposits
- remove gross calculus deposits
- definitive oral examination with charting
- radiographs as required
- supragingival scaling and subgingival scaling (up to 2 mm depth)
- subgingival scaling of pockets over 2 mm and root planing by hand curettes
- check the teeth for residual calculus and remove as found
- tooth extractions
- polish
- subgingival lavage.

Calculus recording and removal

A full oral/dental examination with charting should be performed before any scaling of the teeth. To allow the teeth to be examined, thick coverings of calculus need to be removed (after having been recorded). Extraction forceps or modified 'calculus forceps', will rapidly crack off large pieces of calculus. Some care needs to be exercised to avoid nipping the gums. Clumsiness could chip a crown, especially on small cat teeth.

Power scaling

Mechanical or powered scalers enable fast and easy removal of calculus. They have a great potential for iatrogenic damage but only when used incorrectly.

Ultrasonic scalers

These are commonly used in veterinary practice. They are called ultrasonic because the scaler tip vibrates at a frequency above hearing range (25 kHz or higher). The tip vibration is generated by a magnostrictive mechanism (e.g. Cavitron) or a piezoelectric mechanism (e.g. Piezon) in the handpiece. The two are comparable in performance but the piezoelectric type has overall advantages despite being more expensive.

In both types, the vibrating tip generates heat and needs to be kept cool by copious water flowing over its entire surface. The water flow rate should be set to give the maximum plume in operation. The magnostrictive types tend to generate more heat and so have greater damage potential.

Both types should be used with a thin pointed tip, sometimes called a perio, sickle or universal insert (e.g. TFI-1000). Inserts or tips designed for subgingival use (e.g. EWPP) are available but cannot be assumed to be safe from causing heat trauma and so should be used with caution. The large (wide) tip is not required as a fine tip will do everything the large one can do and more.

Sonic (air) scalers

Sonic scalers also work with a vibrating tip but at a lower frequency. This means they tend to be less effective but generate less heat and so are safer. Only the best types available (e.g. Densonic or Titan SW) have comparable performance to ultrasonic scalers. They require an air-driven dental unit for operation.

Rotary scalers

Roto pro burs or any other scaling burs should *never* be used. These scaling burs are used in a high-speed dental handpiece to remove calculus rapidly. It is impossible to scale teeth this way without causing severe and irreparable damage to the tooth surface.

Technique for power scalers

The scaler tip moves back and forth in the same plane as the long axis of the handle and so the working (contact) surfaces of the tip are the two sides. These surfaces should be kept in flat contact with the tooth surface – the handle is rotated to adjust the presentation of the tip as the contour of the tooth changes. Generally, the tip is held perpendicularly to the gingival margin and the tooth scaled from the top down (towards the gum). When the teeth are spaced

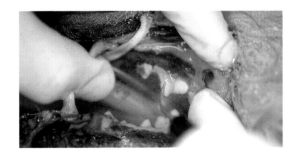

Correct positioning of ultrasonic scaler: the side of the tip is in flat contact with the tooth

it is simple to scale around the entire crown. Where a tooth is in contact with its neighbour, the inter-proximal areas can be scaled by passing the tip horizontally below the contact point.

The scaler will work most efficiently when used with light pressure and continuous small wiping motion. When the calculus is difficult to remove, approach it from different directions and lumps will dislodge. Do not press harder with the scaler as this will suppress the vibration and be self-defeating.

The pointed end of the scaler tip should not be used in contact with the tooth as it will engrave the tooth surface. The damage may not be visible but the surface will be roughened and so more plaque-retentive. There is great temptation to use the point to clean the grooves and fissures of teeth but it is better to use the side of the scaler along the groove.

Preventing heat trauma

Provided that the scaler tip is kept cool, an ultrasonic scaler can be used on a tooth for an indefinite period. Some older machines develop so much heat that the water cannot keep them cool. In that case, the power setting needs to be reduced or the scaler rested periodically.

A hot scaler tip can burn gingival tissues. It can also heat the tooth leading to inflammation of the pulp. This means post-treatment pain. The pulpitis may not resolve and can lead to the pulp becoming necrotic after a prolonged toothache. The risk of pulpitis increases with the contact time of a hot scaler tip. A scaler can be tested by running it on your own finger, as for scaling a tooth.

Remember: copious water cooling and reduce the power setting if the tip is still hot.

When the tip is inserted into a periodontal pocket, it can no longer be cooled by the water as the surface is enclosed by tooth and gingiva. The deeper the tip is inserted, the more quickly the it will become dangerously hot. The simple rule of thumb is that the tip should *never* be used more that 2 mm below the gum line and for only a brief time (less than 2 seconds) before being withdrawn to cool. A simple and accurate test, for each individual scaler, is to pinch the last 2 mm of the tip between thumb and forefinger and see how long it can be held comfortably. The same test should be applied to specialised tips designed for subgingival use.

Hand scaling

All scaling (except when there is a pocket depth over 2 mm) can be achieved with a power scaler. A highly trained operator may claim that scaling can be performed as quickly or better by hand scaling instruments. However, most people would prefer to use hand scalers for only small amounts of scaling or as a temporary measure when the power scaler needs repair.

All dental instruments – including dental handpieces but excluding extraction instruments – should be held in a modified pen grip (Figure 10, overleaf). This is as one would hold a pen but with the middle finger extended to be against the instrument close to its end and the ring finger forming a finger rest.

The only type of hand scaler required is a double-ended sickle pattern (Figure 11, overleaf). The sickle-shaped ends conform to the contour of the tooth. The two ends form a pair: left and right curvature. The working part of the instrument is called the toe and has two sharp

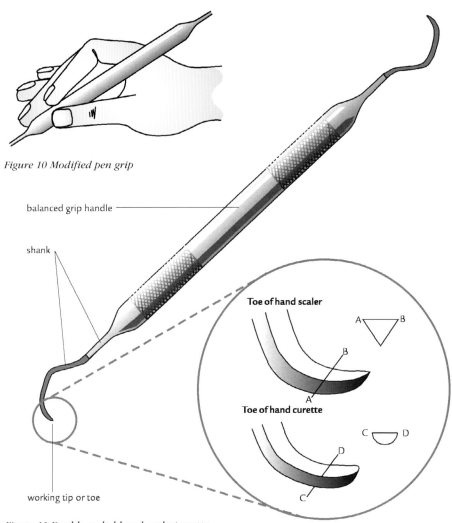

Figure 10 Modified pen grip

balanced grip handle

shank

Toe of hand scaler

A B

B

A

Toe of hand curette

C D

D

C

working tip or toe

Figure 11 Double-ended hand scaler/curette

edges and a flat top. The flat top is kept at 90° to the tooth surface so that the sharp edge contacts the tooth and the flat surface is against the calculus. The hand scaler should be placed on the tooth at or just under the gum line and scraped over the crown away from the gum.

Curettes

A dental curette is a modified hand scaler for use below the gum line (Figure 11). The toe is smaller to fit more easily into the periodontal pocket. The end and back of the toe are rounded, as opposed to sharp, to reduce soft tissue trauma.

Curettes are required to scale the root surfaces in pockets deeper than 2 mm. The technique is similar to that used with a hand scaler but is performed blind and with the constraint of the overlying gingiva. Perfecting hand scaling on the crown should precede using a curette in periodontal pockets.

Root planing

In addition to removing all calculus from the root surfaces, the curette is also used to remove the cementum from the root in a periodontal pocket. The scraping away of this necrotic and infected cementum to leave a smooth healthy root surface is called root planing.

To work effectively, the scalers and curettes must be kept with sharp edges and need re-sharpening after every few uses. They are sharpened by running the toe over a fine, oiled sharpening stone in the same manner as if scaling a tooth.

Checking scaling

The mouth should be scaled systematically so surfaces of teeth are not missed. Begin at the central incisor and scale successive teeth to the back of the mouth. Only surfaces with calculus deposits need to be scaled. When a section of scaling is complete, it should be checked by rinsing and drying the teeth with the 3-in-1 syringe. After drying with compressed air, any remaining specks of calculus are much more visible. The airstream also lifts the gum margin to allow checking of the gingival sulcus and pockets. Alternatively, the sulcus can be checked by sliding the side of a probe over the tooth.

Checking for residual calculus can also be done with a disclosing solution to stain the plaque. After scaling, disclosing solution is swabbed over the teeth, using a cotton bud. The excess solution is rinsed off and the remaining stained plaque also highlights residual calculus deposits.

Tooth extractions

It is sometimes recommended that extractions be carried out at the end of dental treatment, when the mouth is clean, so reducing the risk of contamination of the socket.

Alternatively, extractions are performed after scaling and before polishing. After the extractions, the depth of anaesthesia can be reduced as the remaining treatment is not painful. Having done the extractions, the remaining teeth can be better checked and final scaling and polishing performed more efficiently. The mouth can be rinsed prior to extractions to remove gross debris. The sockets fill with blood clot rapidly and are unlikely to trap subsequent debris.

Polishing

The aim of polishing is to make the tooth surface smooth and, therefore, less plaque-retentive; it will subsequently be easier to maintain plaque-free with home care. Polishing smoothes out microscopic scratches and removes small flecks of calculus (which would otherwise act as centres for formation of new calculus). Polishing also removes plaque and surface stain.

Removing stain is purely a cosmetic benefit. A coarse polishing paste removes stain more effectively but scours the surface. Generally, a fine paste should be used to ensure the surface is actually polished. If a coarse paste is used, it should be followed by a fine paste to smooth out the scratches.

Polishing is done using a dental handpiece with a rubber cup (or brush). Any other method is futile. The rubber cup should not be too stiff; light pressure should flatten and flare the cup edge.

The benefits of polishing are minimal if not followed up with home care.

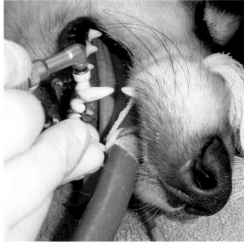

Polishing a crown

Technique for polishing

Keep the polisher at a constant low speed: do not stop and start. Pick up some polishing paste and apply the polisher to the tooth with a light pressure. Move the cup over all the crown and then allow the cup to nudge back the gum margin with the flared edge going a short distance beneath the gum. Do not allow the polisher to over run on top of the gum as it will remove epithelium and leave a raw area. The teeth are polished in a systematic way, as for scaling.

Use plenty of paste to help polishing and to reduce the frictional heat. The paste should be decanted into a small container (such as a Dappens dish) to avoid contamination of the other paste.

Preventing heat trauma

Dental polishers have a very high potential for generating heat by friction of the polisher against the tooth. Higher rotational speed and greater pressure increases the friction and the heat generated. The potential for damage to the pulp is great: incorrect polishing can put much heat into the tooth — considerably more than by misuse of a power scaler. The speed needs to be restricted to the low rate of 4000 rpm. This is easier with a micromotor dental unit as the speed control can be set. On air-driven units, the speed is reduced by part-pressing the foot pedal or reducing the air flow by adjusting the collar below the air motor.

To ensure that your technique is safe, you should use exactly the same technique on your own tooth or finger nail. There is no feedback from an anaesthetised animal; no way of assessing if you have caused toothache or worse. Be aware.

Flush and irrigate pockets

The final part of dental treatment is to rinse the mouth, preferably with 0.2% chlorhexidine solution. Periodontal pockets are irrigated with the same solution using a syringe with a blunt-ended, side-exiting (endodontic) needle. A 20 g hypodermic needle can be modified, using a dental drill, by cutting off the sharp end and creating a slot in the end.

Fluoride application

There is no indication for topical fluoride application as part of dental treatment in animals. Animal fluoride preparations are available, with recommendation to apply at the end of dental treatment, but these have no proven benefit and considerable potential for harm.

Periodontal surgery

Minor periodontal surgery

Resection of gingival hyperplasia to remove false pocketing is part of routine periodontal therapy. The gingivectomy (or rather partial gingival removal) can be done with a scalpel or electrocautery loop. The aim is to return the gingival margin to the normal position. Sometimes more gingiva can be removed to reduce the actual pocket depth but at least a 3 mm band of attached gingiva must remain. Care must be taken not to cut below the attachment level so removing too much tissue.

Open curettage

Reflecting a gingival flap allows direct vision and access to the root surfaces above bone. This enables better and easier treatment of these areas. This approach is only to be considered when the owners have proven an excellent standard of home care.

Advanced periodontal surgery

More advanced forms of periodontal surgery require specialist training but will only achieve benefits when combined with long-term 'gold standard' home care. In the animal patient, true periodontal surgery is to be considered only rarely.

Antibiotics

Antibiotic therapy is not part of routine periodontal disease treatment. Antibiotics are indicated for specific situations associated with periodontal disease and its treatment, but are not used for treatment of the disease itself. Pulse (antibiotic) therapy has recently been proposed as a part of periodontal disease management but has not gained support by specialist periodontists. A major concern is that by inappropriate and over-use of antibiotics, the situation is made worse as competition from less harmful bacteria is reduced and the pathogenic bacteria may become resistant.

Indications for antibiotic use

Antibiotics should be used only when there is an actual requirement in the treatment or they are thought to be necessary as a prophylactic measure.

Antibiotics should only be used prior to dental treatment when there is significant infection, which is causing pain or compromising general health, and there are factors delaying the provision of treatment. Antibiotics prior to treatment have been recommended to reduce the bacterial reservoir in the mouth making treatment safer and improve healing. This can be better achieved by flushing the mouth with chlorhexidine before treatment.

It is known that scaling and extracting teeth results in a bacteraemia. The more severe the periodontal disease, the greater the level of bacteraemia. The bacteraemia can have knock-on adverse effects at other organ sites. When there are known or suspected general health problems, especially renal or cardiac, antibiotic cover during treatment is indicated. The optimum circulating antibiotic concentration at time of procedure is best achieved by administration by injection.

Treatment alone is usually sufficient to give resolution and antibiotics are not routinely required. Generally, the mouth heals very well mainly due to its excellent blood supply. Antibiotics should be considered for animals with known or suspected concomitant problems that may reduce normal healing capability (e.g. immune-compromised patients and those on long-term steroid therapy).

6 Dental diagnosis: indications for tooth extraction

When examining each tooth, a decision needs to be made as to whether or not treatment is required. The tooth may have some abnormality but still be healthy. When there is significant pathology (with associated pain or infection), treatment should be performed as soon as possible. Other pathology may be detected, which may not have associated pain or infection at that time but is certain to progress, and this should be treated sooner rather than later.

The majority of dental pathology can be treated by tooth extraction. This is usually the simple and predictable option. There maybe an alternative treatment that will return the tooth to a satisfactory state of health. Extraction is always preferable to 'supervised neglect' or non-treatment of pathology.

Indications for extraction are:

- periodontal disease
- relief of tooth crowding and retained deciduous teeth
- tooth resorption – feline odontoclastic resorptive lesions (FORLs), lesions in the dog
- fractured teeth – crown or root
- luxation (loosening) – with possible alveolar fracture
- pulp necrosis (trauma, iatrogenic damage)
- traumatic 'bite' (malocclusion)
- caries (tooth decay)
- feline gingivo-stomatitis
- ectopic, un-erupted or impacted teeth
- failed restorative treatment.

Periodontal disease

Periodontal disease is the greatest cause of tooth loss in cats and dogs. As periodontal disease progresses, the local environment becomes more conducive to disease progression and so control of the disease by whatever treatment becomes more difficult. A point comes when the battle is lost and the best interest of the patient is served by extracting the tooth rather than allowing the inevitable progression to advanced stage disease with its potential health implications and pain.

A combination of many factors determines the prognosis of a tooth with periodontal disease. Deepest periodontal pocket depth is the main parameter in assigning prognosis. Pocket depth alone could be used in deciding when to extract but other factors should be considered and the decision point may be moderated. Some of these other factors are:

- the amount of remaining bone support
- the level of on going oral hygiene maintenance

- the age of the animal
- the overall condition of the mouth.

A periodontal pocket greater than 5 mm at a tooth is considered a poor prognosis; extraction should be considered. In the canine teeth, the limit may be increased to 7 mm on the buccal aspect. The limit is scaled down for cats (to 2 mm) and the toy/miniature size dogs (under approx. 4 kg).

A pocket that extends into the furcation area of 3-rooted teeth, demonstrated by the periodontal probing passing horizontally

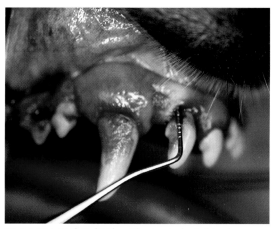

Measuring pocket depth with a periodontal probe

between the roots to under the centre of the crown, means there is a site that is non-amenable to treatment. As prevention of disease is not possible, extraction should be considered. Furcation exposure on 2-rooted teeth does not indicate extraction although it does mean greater stagnation of plaque and food. Extraction of teeth with furcation exposure is to be considered when there is also pocketing and no ongoing tooth brushing.

Relief of tooth crowding and retained deciduous teeth

Tooth crowding can be generalised or localised, where two teeth are in abnormal proximity or overlapped (e.g. lower 4th premolar crowded on the lower carnassial tooth). Extracting teeth

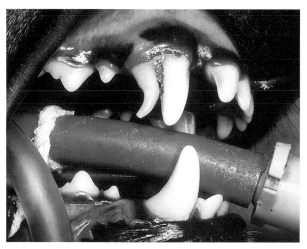

Retained deciduous teeth causing tooth crowding and accumulation of debris

of lesser functional importance will improve the prognosis of the remaining teeth. Crowding results in debris build up between the teeth and greater plaque stagnation, in an area that is less accessible than normal to tooth brushing. This applies to retained deciduous teeth. Even when the tooth positioning is normal, extraction of a tooth may be considered to make its more important neighbour easier to maintain (e.g. lower third incisor in contact with the canine).

Feline odontoclastic resorptive lesions (FORLs)

With the present lack of knowledge of aetiology or associated causal factors, the only treatment option here is extraction. Early diagnosis means easier extraction because as the lesion progresses the tooth becomes more fragile and ankylosis of the root to bone develops. In cats, 25% of animals will have one or more teeth affected by a resorptive lesion. All areas where the gingival margin is hyperplastic or hyperaemic should be investigated for concavities in the underlying tooth surface. The gingiva may initially seem 'stuck' to the tooth. FORLs on the root surfaces can only be detected by radiographs.

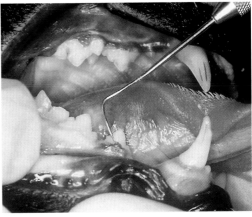

Early FORL (shown by probe) and more advanced lesion on upper carnassial tooth

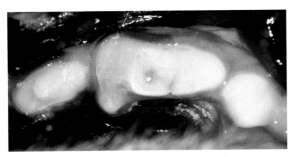

Slab fracture of carnassial tooth with vital pulp exposure

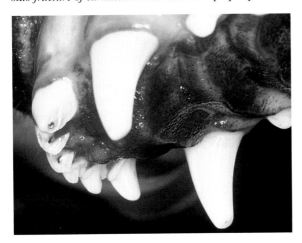

Fractured teeth

Whenever a tooth is fractured so that there is a communication between the pulp and the oral environment, bacteria will enter the pulp. Initially there will be a pulpitis and later pulp necrosis. Fractured crowns should be probed (while the animal is unconscious) to determine whether or not there is an opening to the pulp canal. Fine seeker probes (e.g. Pathfinders) may be useful to detect small exposures. If there is still doubt, a radiograph is indicated. When an opening is found and restorative treatment is not an option, the tooth should always be extracted.

Three fractured incisors with exposed pulp canals and necrotic pulps

Luxation

Trauma can result in loosening of the tooth in the socket, with or without tooth fracture. In some cases, the alveolar bone may be fractured so disrupting one wall of the socket; this is often detected because of a tear in the overlying gingiva. Movement of the tooth, especially in a vertical direction, often results in disruption of the blood supply to the tooth leading to pulp necrosis.

Pulp necrosis

The main sign of pulp necrosis is crown discoloration that is not a surface discoloration. This is due to a release of blood pigments (from the breakdown of pulpal tissue), which diffuse into the porous dentine. Ingress of bacteria is the most common cause of pulp necrosis – the ingress can be secondary to a tooth fracture or a hairline crack (microfracture) or through an advanced carious lesion. Other insults such as heat trauma (iatrogenic damage in polishing or power scaling) can cause a pulpitis that leads to necrosis.

A traumatic force can cause a pulpitis or tooth luxation. Either can lead to pulp necrosis and there is not necessarily any damage to the crown. Teeth with necrotic pulps should be treated. The only exception is necrosis where the root canal is stenosed; this occasionally occurs in larger dogs (usually over eight years old) as a process of ageing.

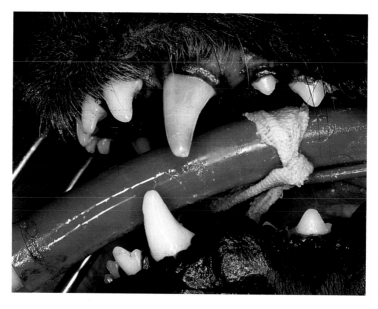

Discoloured crown due to necrotic pulp

Traumatic 'bite' or malocclusion

Tooth malposition or skeletal abnormality can mean that a tooth is positioned so that it makes contact with the soft tissue of the opposite jaw. Unless this contact is very minor and without

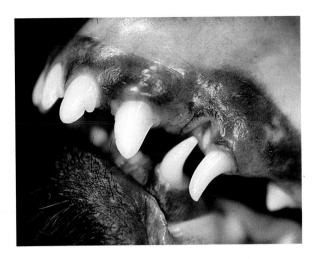

*Traumatic 'bite':
brachygnathic jaw causing
lower (deciduous) canine
tooth to damage soft tissue*

any sign of tissue damage, the problem teeth need treatment: extraction is usually the best option. However, extractions in very young animals can be challenging because the roots are immature and fragile.

Caries (tooth decay)

Tooth decay leading to carious cavities is not uncommon in dogs. It occurs more frequently in larger dogs, especially Rottweillers and Weimaraners. Decay almost always starts in the pits or fissures of the molar teeth. Once the lesion has gone through the enamel and into the dentine, it is irreversible and will only progress if untreated. When a dental explorer penetrates into the tooth surface, and a tug is felt on withdrawal, the lesion needs treatment even if no cavity is obvious. A simple filling may be an easier treatment option for a small cavity but, once the damage is extensive, extraction is the best option.

> **Extraction of certain teeth may be considered difficult. Postponing the extraction only prolongs pain and/or infection for the animal. If in doubt, take it out.**

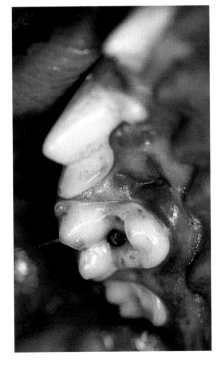

Caries: upper 1st molar

7 Tooth extraction: basic technique

Tooth extraction can be very challenging and is rarely an easy procedure. A successful extraction is when the entire tooth is removed with the minimum of trauma to the adjacent remaining tissues (and the operator). The best success rate is achieved by practitioners who have:

- knowledge of tooth root morphology
- correct technique
- appropriate equipment
- practice and patience.

Root morphology

The operator needs to be familiar with the normal shape and number of roots of all the teeth. Be aware that abnormalities such as extra roots or abnormally shaped roots (e.g. hooks) are not uncommon. For a reminder of normal root pattern, refer to Dentalabels dental charts, Visimodels or a dry skull.

Technique

In cats and dogs, the routine technique for extraction is to loosen (luxate) and extract (elevate) each tooth root individually. The crowns of 2- and 3-rooted teeth need to be sectioned, in all cases, to produce single root pieces prior to extraction. This is required because the roots of multi-rooted teeth are usually divergent and, therefore, have different paths of withdrawal.

Sectioning multi-rooted teeth

Using a dental drill to section the crown enables cutting that is accurate and quick, and causes minimum trauma to adjacent tissues. A small diameter (size 012) fissure bur in a high-speed dental handpiece with water cooling is ideal. Next best is a micromotor-powered dental drill with a fissure bur. Rotating discs, hacksaws etc. should not be used as correct positioning of the cut is difficult, and they cause unnecessary trauma to other tissues.

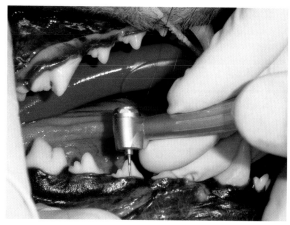

Dental drill with fissure bur (size 012) sectioning a premolar crown

The first step is to locate the furcation. This is generally directly below the main cuspal point of the crown. It is found by feeling for a concavity with a dental probe or by slightly reflecting the gum margin (with an instrument or the air syringe) to see the furcation. The crown is cut beginning near the furcation, just above gum level, from the buccal aspect to the lingual side. The cut is then deepened behind the gum to achieve complete crown division. Test the division by gently wedging an elevator between the sectioned crown and observing slight movement of the crown parts in opposite directions.

Sectioning 3-rooted teeth (upper carnassial teeth and the upper molar teeth in dogs) can only be achieved by using fissure burs in dental handpieces.

Usually, crowns are sectioned by vertical cuts (Figures 12 and 13). In large teeth, the crown height may be greater than the bur length. In these teeth, either the crown is first cut horizontally to reduce its height or the cut is angled to go through the crown where it is less high. This also means less tooth-cutting is needed so sectioning is quicker.

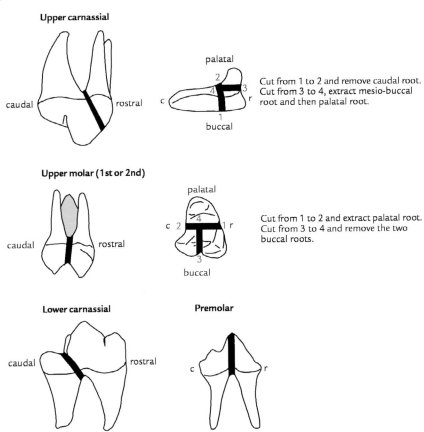

Upper carnassial

palatal

caudal   rostral   c

buccal

Cut from 1 to 2 and remove caudal root.
Cut from 3 to 4, extract mesio-buccal root and then palatal root.

Upper molar (1st or 2nd)

palatal

caudal   rostral   c 2   1 r

buccal

Cut from 1 to 2 and extract palatal root.
Cut from 3 to 4 and remove the two buccal roots.

Lower carnassial   **Premolar**

caudal   rostral   c   r

cut with fissure bur

Figure 12 Sectioning dog teeth: upper carnassial and molar, lower carnassial and premolar

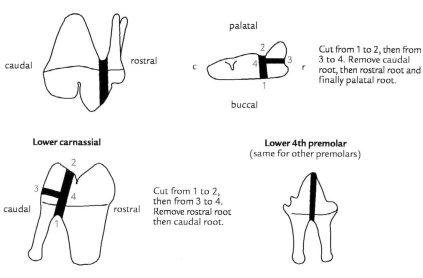

Upper carnassial

palatal

buccal

Cut from 1 to 2, then from 3 to 4. Remove caudal root, then rostral root and finally palatal root.

Lower carnassial

Cut from 1 to 2, then from 3 to 4. Remove rostral root then caudal root.

Lower 4th premolar
(same for other premolars)

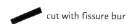 cut with fissure bur

Figure 13 Sectioning cat teeth: upper carnassial, lower carnassial and premolar

Cutting the gingival attachment

As part of severing the tooth's attachment, the gingival attachment of the tooth should be cut around its entire circumference. This can be done by running a scalpel blade around the gingival sulcus or pocket and cutting down the root surface to crestal bone. The gingival attachment can also be cut using a sharp dental elevator when starting luxation. Failure to cut the gingival attachment results in unnecessary disruption and trauma to the soft tissues as the tooth is extracted.

Root luxation

Luxation is the loosening of the tooth in the socket by progressive disruption of the periodontal ligament fibres. A Couplands elevator (or similar instrument) is used. The curvature of the gouge part of the tip should be similar to that of the root surface and so give a close fit. A Couplands No. 1 (3 mm wide) is suitable for most medium-size dogs' teeth. A larger Couplands (No. 2 or 3) is needed for bigger teeth and a Super Slim elevator (2 mm) for cats' teeth.

The elevator is inserted behind the gingiva, at an acute angle to the tooth root, until it hits crestal bone. The instrument tip is then wedged between the root and bone, and gently rotated (not levered) to move the tooth laterally. The pressure is built up gradually and then

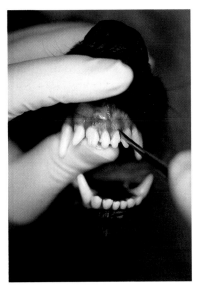

held for five seconds to stretch and break the periodontal fibres. The elevator is then relocated at different sites around the tooth and the procedure repeated until the tooth root becomes loose. Patience and controlled force are needed, not brute strength. The force should be applied as low down the root as possible when extracting teeth. Slipping when using an elevator is often because the tooth moves. You should support the jaw with your other hand and have a thumb and finger either side of the tooth being extracted. Using the dental air/water syringe during extraction to rinse away blood and then keeping it at bay with the air stream enables clear vision thus helping to position the elevator and monitor progress.

Couplands elevator inserted into the gingival sulcus to cut and luxate

Root elevation and extraction

In dogs, the tooth can be extracted by using only the elevator but usually it is simpler to finish the extraction using extraction forceps. Pattern 76N forceps are recommended for all cat teeth and most dog teeth (except large teeth). The final periodontal fibres are broken by slightly rotating the root in the socket. As dogs' teeth roots are neither straight nor round in cross-section, they will not rotate more that a degree or two. When the root will turn a little in both directions, the forceps can be used to pull the tooth from the socket. The beaks of extraction forceps should fit the root and make a 4-point contact. The root should always be gripped as low down as possible to reduce the torque on the root and so reduce the risk of breakage.

In cats, the forceps can be employed earlier and to greater effect to luxate the tooth. Once the root is loosened by the elevator, the forceps can be used to rotate the tooth in the socket. Cats' teeth roots tend to be straight and circular in cross-section and so allow greater rotation. Care should be taken not to crush the tooth with the forceps or to allow forces across the long axis of the root. Feline tooth roots usually have a bulbous end. When the root is quite loose, it is withdrawn by pulling along its long axis and 'popping' the bulbous root-end through the narrower socket above.

Root atomisation

This is not a proper extraction technique and should only be employed as a technique of last choice.

The idea is that the root is drilled out using high speed dental drills. This technique can only be condoned for removal of feline teeth with odontoclastic resorptive lesions when the root is ankylosed or resorbed. It is better to leave a small piece of root tip rather than over-drill and cause damage to adjacent structures such as the inferior alveolar canal or the nasal spaces. There is insufficient follow-up information available to know whether or not this is actually an acceptable procedure.

Equipment

Ideally, extraction kits should be kept prepared and sterilised ready for each situation. Choice of many of the instruments, or the particular pattern of a certain instrument, will be according to the personal preference of the operator. Essential items are listed in Chapter 9 (page 48).

Treatment of the socket

Once the tooth has been extracted, the aim is to promote the best healing of the socket. Sharp bony projections and any loose bone pieces should be removed. Non-viable soft tissue, such as superfluous pieces with dubious blood supply, may also be removed. Granulation tissue should be removed by gently curetting the socket.

Packing or suturing?

It should be considered whether the suturing or packing of a socket aids healing and reduces post op pain or actually hinders healing due to the extra tissue manipulation and the presence of foreign material. Extraction sockets heal very well naturally and the author feels that minimal intervention is best.

In normal healing, the tooth socket will fill with a blood clot and, later, new bone. There is little evidence that any of the bone-like products suggested for use to fill the socket actually give a clinically significant increase in bone in-fill.

Suturing to hold the marginal gingivae in their proper position is indicated where these tissues have become very mobile. Closing the gingiva over a socket may reduce some post-operative pain and ensure blood-clot retention. To allow closure, the gingiva has to be first loosened to enable apposition without tension. This extra handling of the tissues results in trauma and, therefore, pain. Sutures themselves may complicate healing due to tissue reaction and debris trapping. Suturing sockets closed involves significant time and cost and generally provides little benefit.

Gentle and proper extraction technique is the way to achieve best healing and minimise post-extraction pain. The amount of post-operative pain correlates to the degree of trauma to the adjacent bone and soft tissue during extraction.

Extraction difficulties and complications

Extraction may be made more difficult by root abnormalities (e.g. excess curvature or hooks) or root ankylosis.

Ankylosis

A calcific bridge from socket to root is the cause of ankylosis. This is common in cats' teeth with resorptive lesions and also in old dogs with a slowly progressive periodontal disease. When an extraction is attempted and no 'give' is felt in the tooth, ankylosis is the likely reason. A normal extraction technique should be continued in an attempt to breakdown the ankylosis.

If this is not possible, a surgical extraction will be required (or root atomisation on cats' teeth with FORLs).

Complications

Complications usually result from incorrect technique or insufficient care in extraction. They include:

- iatrogenic damage to adjacent tissues
- fractured roots or remnant root tips
- displaced root fragments
- fistula
- dry socket
- jaw fracture
- delayed or complicated healing.

Fractured roots and remnant root tips

The ideal is to avoid this situation by correct technique. Unless the fracture is considerably below bone level, it may still be possible to remove the root remnant by further use of elevators (especially Super Slim) or other instruments. Removal of a small gutter of bone around the top of the root fragment, using a dental drill, can facilitate access with the elevator. Surgical extraction technique allows the removal of any root remnants. A surgical approach may give a better and quicker result especially when the root fragment is deep in the bone.

When can a root fragment be left?

A root fragment cannot be left if it has associated infection or pathology. A tooth that had a necrotic pulp must always be entirely removed. It may be argued that the potential complication from leaving a small piece of previously healthy root tip is sufficiently small that the trauma of entire removal is unjustified. This may be so, but should not be used as a general excuse. Leaving any root remnant may be considered dubious, however small the risk of complication, because of the lack of follow-up possible for an animal. When a root piece remains, a check radiograph should be taken and the animal's records clearly marked to indicate its position. Follow-up radiographs should be obtained at future anaesthetic procedures, in case of developing pathology.

Displaced root fragments

When trying to remove a root remnant, especially the palatal root or the upper carnassial tooth or feline mandibular premolar roots, care should be taken to avoid downwards force that may push the root through the base of the socket. The root piece is then very difficult to retrieve and can cause problems.

Fistula

An oro-nasal fistula can result after extracting a maxillary tooth. The upper canine tooth in dogs is the most common site. When there is long-standing infection on the medial aspect, a fistula may be pre-existing and removal of the tooth 'unplugs' the defect. Extraction of the upper canine can easily disrupt the bone septum between the socket and nasal cavity, and may tear the nasal epithelium. This may heal or form a persistent fistula. This unnecessary complication can be avoided by using a surgical extraction technique.

Dry socket

This is a well-recognised condition in humans and leads to a marked increase in pain about three days after extraction. It is associated with loss of clot from the socket and exposure of the bony surface. It is more common after difficult extractions when greater forces are used and more trauma is caused. In humans, the socket is cleaned and packed with an obtundant and antiseptic dressing.

Dry socket is thought to occur in animals where signs of pain and possibly pyrexia may be noticed a few days after the dental extraction. Treatment is with antibiotics.

Post-extraction care

Advice to feed soft food, which is more likely to stick in the sockets, can be counter-productive. Normal food should be given. Only if difficulty is perceived should softer, but *not* sticky, food (e.g. flaked fish or cooked chicken) be given.

Oral hygiene methods should be recommenced immediately. Topical application of chlorhexidine preparations could be substituted for a short period if there is an objection to tooth brushing. Tough chew toys should be withheld for about a week when sutures have been placed.

Analgesia should be given prior to extraction(s) and additional follow-up analgesia considered. The amount of pain depends on the difficulty of the extraction, the number of extraction sites and the individual patient.

Antibiotics

A course of antibiotics is not routinely indicated after tooth extraction. Removal of the offending tooth provides sufficient surgical drainage for an infection site. However, the presence of osteomyelitis does require antibiotic therapy, which may be used both pre- and post-operatively.

Antibiotics are used when there is a specific reason for their requirement. Pre–extraction antibiotic cover is indicated to protect against the resultant bacteraemia in cases with known or suspected underlying medical problems. Renal conditions and cardiac conditions (with impaired endothelium) especially require cover.

Post-operative antibiotics should be considered for animals that have impaired healing capability (e.g. immune-compromised animals, animals on long-term steroid therapy).

8 Tooth extraction: surgical technique

A surgical extraction technique, or open extraction technique, is indicated for removal of all canine teeth and root fragments. Some people prefer this approach for the extraction of multiple adjacent teeth and deciduous teeth. A surgical extraction involves raising a gingival flap, then removing some of the bone that forms the tooth socket so facilitating the extraction. The following description is of the extraction of an upper canine tooth in a dog. All teeth can be extracted by making minor modifications to this technique.

Surgical technique

The gingival flap

The flap is outlined with basic surgical principles in mind. The incisions should be over bone that will not be removed during the procedure. The base of the flap (towards the buccal sulcus) should be broader than the edge – the blood supply to the flap is only through its base as the periosteal supply will be disrupted. The flap should be made large enough from the outset to give generous access.

Incisions

The incisions (Figure 14) are made with a pointed tip scalpel (No. 15 on No. 11) held in a handle. The incisions need to be made forcefully to cut the full thickness, including the periosteum, and score the bone. A incision is made along the crestal ridge of the alveolar bone

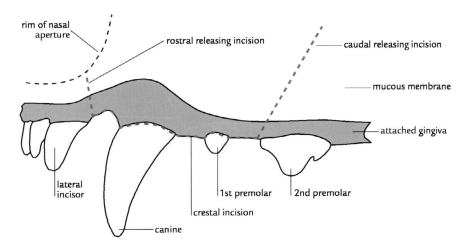

Figure 14 Outline of incisions to raise gingival flap: upper canine tooth

beginning just distal (caudal) to the lateral incisor tooth up to the mesial point of the canine, continuing around the buccal gingival sulcus, along to the 1st premolar, around the buccal sulcus of the 1st premolar and almost to the mesial (rostral) aspect of the 2nd premolar. A rostral releasing incision is made from the rostral end of the crestal incision extending towards the sulcus across the attached gingiva but stopping before the bony rim of the nasal aperture. A longer caudal releasing incision is also made. It is useful to go over the incisions several times and in opposite directions to ensure they are complete.

Raising the flap

The full thickness, mucoperiosteal flap is peeled back using a periosteal elevator. A Goldman-Fox or Molt periosteal elevator is a popular choice. Begin at the caudal corner. The sharp end of the elevator needs to get under the periosteum but the instrument should be held at an obtuse angle so that the back of the instrument pushes the soft tissue and keeps it as one sheet. If the instrument is too low (acute angle) it will tend to split through the tissue layers. The attached gingiva is difficult to raise but once beyond the mucogingival junction, the flap reflects easily. Once reflected, the flap is held away to avoid trauma.

Bone removal

The outline of the root can be seen as the overlying bone is raised. The apex of the canine root is in line with the rostral root of the 2nd premolar. Using a dental drill, a line of bone is removed to expose the root and then further bone is removed in a direction towards the edge

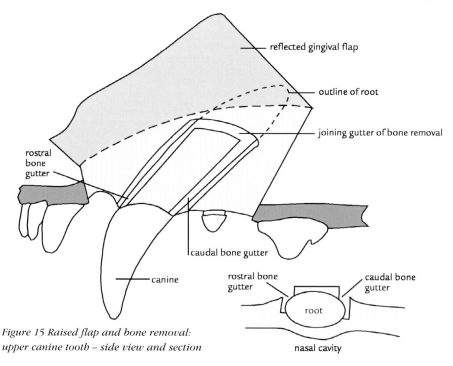

Figure 15 Raised flap and bone removal:
upper canine tooth – side view and section

of the root. When the edge of the root is located, a narrow gutter is made from the crest (near the gum margin) along two-thirds of the root length. This is repeated for the other side (caudal or rostral) of the tooth. The gutters need to be deep enough to uncover the widest part of the root but not so deep as to encounter the nasal cavity. The two gutters are connected with a line of bone removal across the root surface (Figure 15).

Copious water cooling is required at all times when drilling bone. Bone is very heat sensitive and a rise of 10 °C can complicate healing.

Luxation and extraction

Once the bone has been removed over three sides for two-thirds of the root length, the remaining periodontal ligament attachment needs to be broken down. Use a Couplands elevator (usually No. 3), alternately in the rostral and caudal gutters, to break the attachment on the medial side.

Once the tooth is loosened, the apical attachment is broken using extraction forceps. The tooth can now be extracted in the direction of the root curvature. To minimise the risk of rupturing the bone septum between socket and nasal cavity, elevator forces are not applied in a lateral or medial direction. Sometimes, this bone can still be torn as the periodontal ligaments are stronger than the bone, and a piece of bone is seen attached to the root. If the nasal epithelium is torn, an ipsilateral nostral bleed is seen. Complete closure with the buccal flap will still allow healing to occur without risk of fistula.

In contrast, for the lower canine extraction, the elevators are *not* placed in the rostral or caudal gutters as this will put stress across the weakest part of the mandible and risk mandibular fracture. The elevators are used on the medial side to wedge against the whole rostral mandible and tip the tooth laterally.

In lower canine extraction, the labial frenulum is cut and raised with the flap and care is taken to avoid the vessels emerging from the mental foramen when reflecting the base of the flap.

Closure

Prior to closure, any loose or sharp bone is removed with the drill or rongeurs. The flap is laid back in its original position. Sutures are placed at each corner (junction of crestal and releasing incision) and then along the releasing incisions. The crestal incision is closed by sutures between the teeth and across the socket. Full closure of the socket is usually possible without any tissue tension. If not, a gap should be left.

Gingiva is very tough but also tears readily. A swaged-on cutting need should be used to avoid tearing. A resorbable, preferably monofilament suture is used (1.5 metric (4/0) is recommended).

Post-operative care

A five day post–operative course of antibiotics is usually given as a prophylactic measure. This may not be necessary but cancellous bone has been opened up. Analgesics are given pre- and post-op as with all extractions. Chew toys are withheld for five days to avoid tearing of the flap or sutures.

9 Dental equipment and supplies

'A bad workman blames his tools' – but a proficient worker has the right tools.

There are certain essential instruments that are necessary to perform basic dentistry in small-animal practice and some further equipment may make these tasks easier.

Most of the equipment required is the same as that used in human dentistry but the range of instruments required is much smaller. A full dental catalogue can be bewildering. Dental instruments have evolved with new designs and improvements but unfortunately the out-dated patterns often seem to end up in veterinary practices.

The essential equipment required for everyday dentistry for cats and dogs is as outlined below. This is not an exhaustive list and does not include items that would already be found in a veterinary practice.

Oral examination

- dental explorer or probe (right-angle straight type, pattern No. 6)
- periodontal or pocket measuring probe (recommended pattern is No. 14 Williams B)
- dental charts (Dentalabels is the best design) – separate feline and canine
- fine seeker probes (Pathfinders, manufactured by Kerr) – an optional item but very useful in determining very small pulp canal exposures in fractured teeth

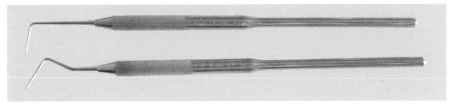

Explorer probe No. 6 (top) and Williams B periodontal probe No. 14 (bottom); instruments from Big-O range

Tooth scaling

Mechanical scalers

Ultrasonic scalers

- piezoelectric type (EMS Piezon or Satelec) with the fine scaler tip (perio/universal/sickle)

or

- magnostrictive type (Cavitron or Bobcat) with the fine scaler tip (perio/universal/sickle)

Air (sonic) scalers

- only consider the best available (e.g. Densonic or Titan SW) – which are also the most expensive

Hand instruments

- hand curettes with balanced grip handles (Columbia 4L/4R or Columbia 13/14) – for fine subgingival scaling and root planing

Curettes are the only instruments to use for scaling deep pockets (over 3 mm) and root planing. Mechanical scalers can not safely be used in deep pockets.

- hand scalers of the sickle or universal type (hygienist pattern H6/H7)

Scalers are used in pairs – left- and right-handed. Hand scalers are for scaling above the gum line. There is little use for hand scalers if you have a mechanical scaler with the correct tip.

- calculus forceps, optional – to crack off large pieces of calculus
- sharpening kit – all hand curettes and scalers must be regularly sharpened

Tooth polishing

- polishing (rubber) cups or brushes – soft type
- polishing paste of a fine grade
- Dappens dishes or other suitable container for single portion of polishing paste
- dental polishing handpiece driven by

  (a) air motor on an air-driven dental unit

  or

  (b) micromotor unit – electric hand motor and control unit

Air-driven dental unit or micromotor unit?

The purchase cost of an air-driven dental unit is about three times that of a micromotor unit but it will do considerably more and last much longer in service. An air-driven dental unit will pay for itself in a very short time. Once you have used one, you will not willingly go back to performing dentistry with out it.

The air-turbine drill has integral water spray to cool the burs and cutting site, and is considerably quicker than a slow handpiece. A slow handpiece is required for polishing and the air motor that drives this is far more robust but it does not have as good speed control as a micromotor.

Air-driven dental units also have a 3-in-1 (air and water) syringe which is very useful for rinsing and drying to aid visibility, especially useful for seeing what is happening during tooth extraction.

Tooth extraction

Sectioning teeth

- fissure bur (usually size 012 or 702) and a smaller fissure bur for cats (size 010 or 701) in

  (a) air turbine dental handpiece (fast)

  or

  (b) contra-angled handpiece with latch grip head (slow)

Elevators

- Couplands No. 1 – for most teeth in dogs (No. 3 may be required for large dog teeth)
- Super Slim elevators – similar to a half-size Couplands – are used for cats and the toy/miniature breeds of dog; also very useful for removing root tips
- periosteal elevator (Goldman-Fox pattern)

Forceps

- upper narrow root forceps (pattern 76N) – for most dog teeth and all cat teeth

- upper incisor forceps (pattern 76) – for larger dog teeth including canines

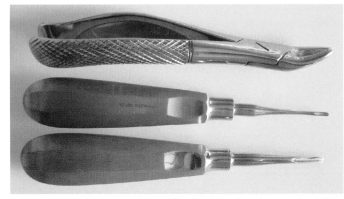

76N extraction forceps (top), Couplands Super Slim elevator (middle) and Couplands No.1 elevator (bottom); instruments from Big-O range

Dental radiography

- a dental X-ray machine is ideal – especially when conveniently placed at the dental treatment table – but a standard veterinary X-ray machine can be used
- small size non-screen X ray film

(a) standard dental film – available in three sizes: occlusal (approx. 5.5 x 7 cm), adult periapical (approx. 3 x 4 cm), paediatric periapical (approx. 2 x 3.5 cm)

Dental film is commonly available in two speeds: D (ultra) and E (ekta). Film designated E is twice as fast as film designated D; it requires less exposure time (radiation dose), but with a small loss of quality.

Veterinary automatic processors can not handle these small films. Standard dental film is processed manually in a 4-bath system in a darkroom, or in a chairside light-safe box. A coffee mug makes an ideal bath. To save time, Kodak's Rapid Access developer and fixer solutions can be used. Alternatively, a dental automatic processor can be purchased.

(b) monoprocessor film – available only in adult periapical size

Monoprocessor film uses a single developer/fixer solution. In some (e.g. ECO-30), the solution is contained in a separate compartment within the film package. The film is processed (in its package) by breaking the seal between the two compartments; thus, no dark facility is required. The film must be thoroughly rinsed immediately after the package is opened. ECO-30 gives comparable quality to standard dental film.

Ancillary supplies

- gloves, face masks and safety specs
- home care products (toothbrushes and toothpaste)
- chlorhexidine gluconate solution 0.2% (e.g. Corsodyl from GlaxoSmithKline)
- endodontic irrigation needles and syringes – to flush deep pockets
- dental mouth mirror (No. 3, small) – also useful as retractors
- mouth props – can be made from sturdy needle caps

Suggested further reading

BSAVA Manual of Small Animal Dentistry (1995)
edited by D A Crossley and S Penman
published by British Small Animal Veterinary Association
ISBN 0-905214-28-5

Small Animal Dentistry (1993)
C Harvey and P Emily
published by Mosby
ISBN 0-8016-6067-9

Veterinary Dentistry: Principles and Practice (1997)
edited by R B Wiggs and H B Lobprise
published by Lippincott–Raven
ISBN 0-397-51385-2

Glossary of common dental terms

Alveolar Pertaining to the alveolus.

Alveolus The more superficial part of the jaw bone (mandible or maxilla), which forms the sockets of the teeth.

Buccal The aspect (of the tooth or other oral structure) towards the cheek.

Distal The aspect of the tooth farthest away from the centre line of the jaw when tracing a line along the dental arch (line of the teeth). The same as the caudal aspect for posterior teeth.

Furcation Forking or branching point. The place under the crown of a tooth where the roots meet or first join together.

Halitosis Abnormal odour of the breath, usually unpleasant.

Lingual The aspect (of the tooth or other oral structure) towards the tongue.

Malocclusion An abnormality of occlusion or jaw/tooth relationship.

Mesial The aspect of the tooth nearest to the centre line of the jaw when tracing a line along the dental arch (line of the teeth). The same as the rostral aspect on posterior (cheek) teeth but not necessarily so for anterior teeth.

Occlusion The 'bite' or the relationship of the upper and lower teeth when the jaws are closed.

Palatal The aspect (of the tooth or other oral structure) towards the palate.

NOTES

NOTES